Beginner's Keto

Learn the Benefits of Ketosis and Why It Is So Popular

Ron Kness

Disclaimer

Copyright © 2019 Ron Kness - All rights reserved.

By reading this document, the reader agrees that under no circumstances are we responsible for any losses, direct or indirect, which are incurred as a result of the use of information contained within this document, including, but not limited to, —errors, omissions, or inaccuracies.

This book is for **personal use only**.

ISBN: 9781796856316

Contents

Introduction

You're tired of looking at yourself in the mirror and pinching the flab around your waist. You're tired of telling yourself that you'll start your diet on Monday… or at the beginning of the month… or on a date that's a nice round number, but never seems to come.

You know you're overweight. You know you want to lose the excess fat… BUT you also know that you've gone down this path before.

You've tried the diet pills. You've gone to the gym for a while. You've tried all the fads and advice that you've read online… and no matter what you do, the weight never seems to come off, or if it does it comes back on and more.

After a month of struggle, at most you've lost a pound or two. To make matters worse, the moment you indulge in some food you love, the pounds return with a vengeance and you're back at square one.

You're tired of this never-ending cycle of planning to lose weight… trying… succeeding a little… and failing. You're tired of ALL of it.

You're probably tired just reading this…

But guess what?

It can all change today … if you want it to!

By the time you've completed this book you'll have all the knowledge you need to lose weight safely in the fastest possible time.

No starving yourself. No hours of mindlessly pounding on the treadmill.

And most importantly – no landing back at square one just because you slip up now and then.

21-Day Challenge

As a bonus, I would like to offer you our **21-Day Keto Challenge**. Just go to https://forms.aweber.com/form/88/537832688.htm to sign up and get started today. Each day of the challenge you will get an email with a task to do for that day and the action steps required to complete it. It helps you stay on track with your Keto diet.

Welcome to the Ketogenic diet – it's not hard…and it's definitely one that can get your great results.

What is Ketosis?

Throughout the years, we've been told that for our bodies to function correctly we need carbohydrates (glucose). What most don't know is that there's a better source of energy called ketones which are produced while you're in ketosis.

Ketosis is the metabolic state your body puts itself into when there is no more glucose left in your body.

When there's no glucose to burn, the body goes straight to the stubborn fat stores and uses the fat for fuel. This is the core principle of the ketogenic diet and is the reason why it's one of the most powerful weight loss protocols on the planet.

Your body is literally emptying your vault of fat and filling it up with ketones which is uses as energy. Weight loss becomes automatic and much easier than if you were to use conventional diets.

How Does It Work?

One of the reasons obesity is an epidemic is because our diets are high in carbohydrates and sugar. Processed carbs get converted into glucose by the body.

Glucose is sugar. In other words, you're giving your body a ton of sugar if your carb consumption is high.

The human body is incapable of burning fat if there is too much glucose in the blood.

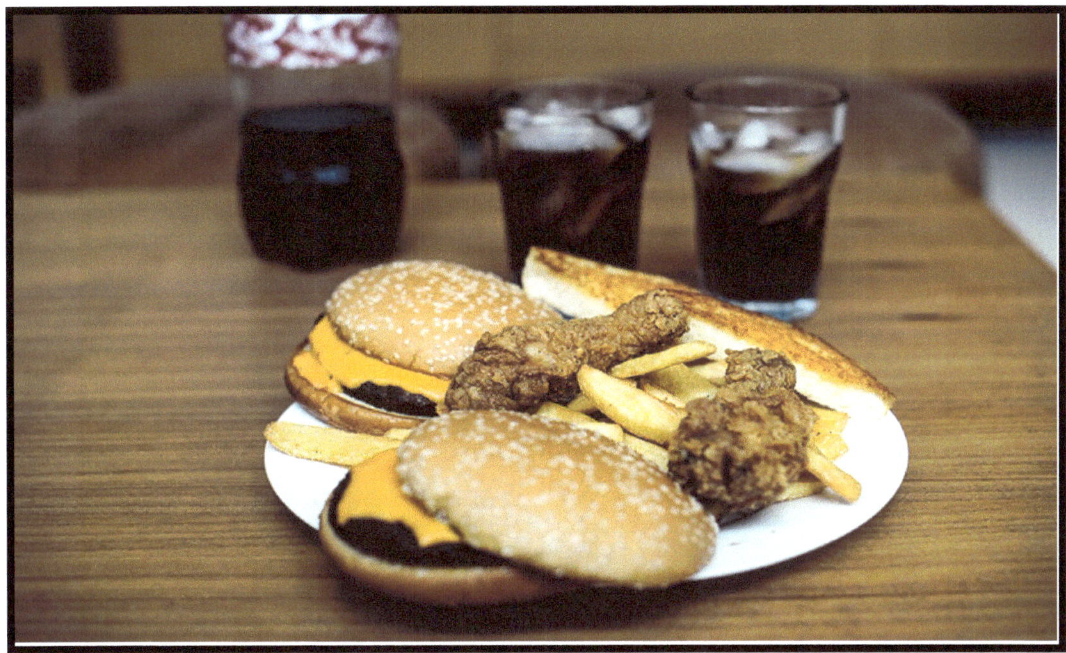

When you're on the keto diet, most of your calories will be in the form of fat. Your carb intake will be very low. This is one of the rules of the keto diet.

Since your diet is low in carbs, your body will be forced to find another source of fuel – your fats. Now the fat burning process begins and accelerates over time.

When you eat less carbs while burning fat, your liver takes fatty acids and turns them in to ketones which will be used as the energy source instead of glucose.

There are three types of ketones:

1. Acetoacetate (AcAc) – This is the first ketone to be created.

2. β-hydroxybutyrate (BHB) – This is created from acetoacetate.

3. Acetone which is created as a side product of acetoacetate

These three ketones will supply you with enough energy to get through day.

In a nutshell, glucose is your main source of energy when you are eating foods with plenty of carbohydrates and when you starve your body of them you enter ketosis.

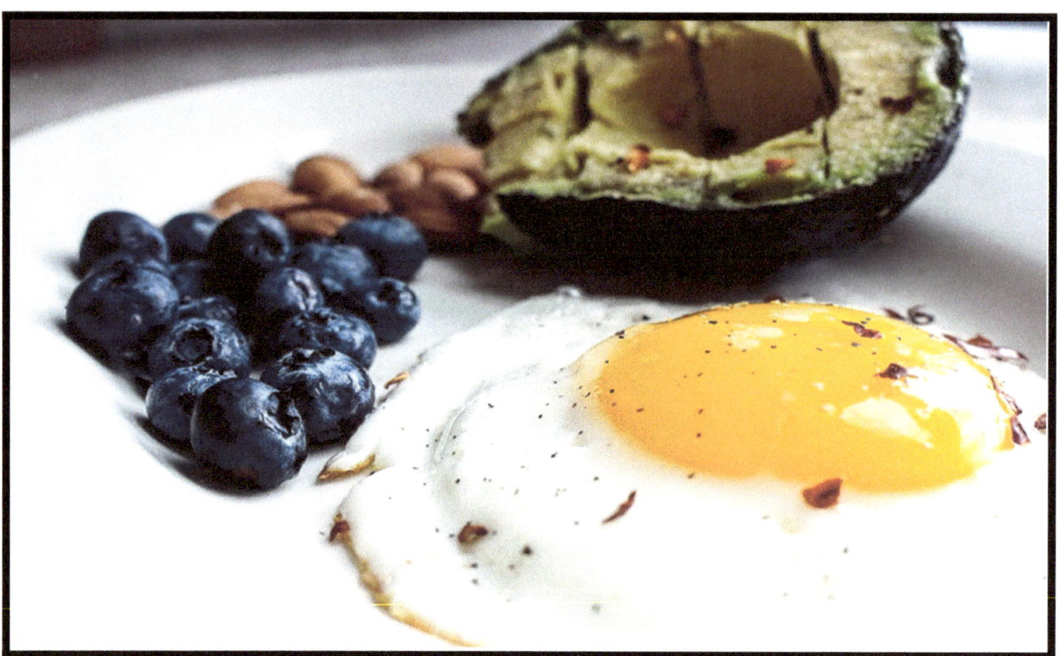

A Quick Overview of the Ketogenic Diet

Now with all of that out the way, here is what we will cover in Beginner's Keto.

You will learn what the benefits of ketosis are and why people are going mad about it.

High profile boxers like Tyson Fury have used ketosis to lose up to 140lbs for his fight on the 3rd November 2018. (Google it…it is an amazing testimonial of the keto diet.)

One hormone that can influence whether or not you get into ketosis is insulin. We will go over how it can help you get into ketosis.

Ketosis is what you want to achieve to start burning weight, <u>but ketoacidosis is what you need to avoid at all costs</u>.

Getting your body ready to burn fat is a process. You have to learn to fine tune your body to get the best out of keto adaption.

Those are just the basics. Next, we are going to dive into actually achieving ketosis and this will be the most challenging part of your journey.

Don't panic. It's still easier than most of the other diets out there.

There are simple strategies and also more advanced strategies you can follow to get into ketosis. It's best that you set goals to help you achieve the results you're striving for.

A superficial understanding of the keto diet will trip you up. Many people believe that they know what to eat and end up falling into a trap of eating foods that they think are good, but in reality, they're sabotaging their weight loss progress.

There's a saying that abs are made in the kitchen. It's very true. More than 80% of your success when it comes to losing weight will rest on the effectiveness of your keto diet.

The remaining 20% is in exercising and getting sufficient rest. Too many people make the cardinal mistake of trying to out exercise a poor diet. You can't do it. Period.

You MUST have your diet dialed in, and then you'll not need to torture yourself at the gym. The weight will still come off, probably faster and more easily.

While on the keto diet your body may start to ache, you will feel hungry and may experience lethargy. All this is normal and temporary.

In this book, you'll learn how to deal with keto-flu and what steps to take to recover and carry on progressing.

Measuring Ketosis

There are three ways to ascertain if you're in ketosis.

1. Using keto sticks
2. Using a breathalyzer
3. Using a ketometer.

Do note that you don't need to test yourself every single day. Later on, we'll cover when it is best to test yourself to see if you are still in ketosis.

We'll also look at intermittent fasting which is extremely powerful for weight loss. When combined with the keto diet, you'll become a fat-burning incinerator and reach your ideal weight in no time at all.

Not a lot of people are guided correctly on how to begin intermittent fasting. You'll learn some of the best techniques here that are being used by people all over the world.

Knowing just a little about intermittent fasting will set you up for great success. Once you are ready, we will then move onto the quickest way getting into ketosis.

There are different strategies that you can follow to get into ketosis quickly and we will show you the best proven way that you can adapt to suit your needs and lifestyle.

Let's get started. We have much to cover and it's all exciting stuff.

Basics of Ketosis

In this chapter, we'll discuss why you need to get into ketosis, and what benefits can be derived from it. Besides giving your brain and body unlimited energy which results in higher physical and mental endurance, there are several other benefits too.

Benefits of Ketosis

You may have a different agenda but here are the best benefits according to research as to why people go into ketosis.

1. Weight loss

Ketosis is all about burning fat, and since the hormone insulin is so low, you'll burn fat at a much higher rate.

You'll feel less hungry, but still have an appetite. While you'll need to cut out most carbohydrate foods, you'll still be able to enjoy fatty foods like bacon.

The keto diet is not as harsh as the paleo diet. There is some degree of flexibility and you can still eat a lot of the fatty foods you love.

It was mentioned earlier how boxer Tyson Fury lost 140 pounds with the keto diet. The man was a walking fat burning machine and eating burger patties as part of this diet.

He wasn't starving or struggling to eat bland, boring foods. That's one of the benefits of the keto diet. You won't have to sacrifice your taste buds. Eating can still be fun.

Once you have ketosis activated and eat the right foods – the weight will drop off.

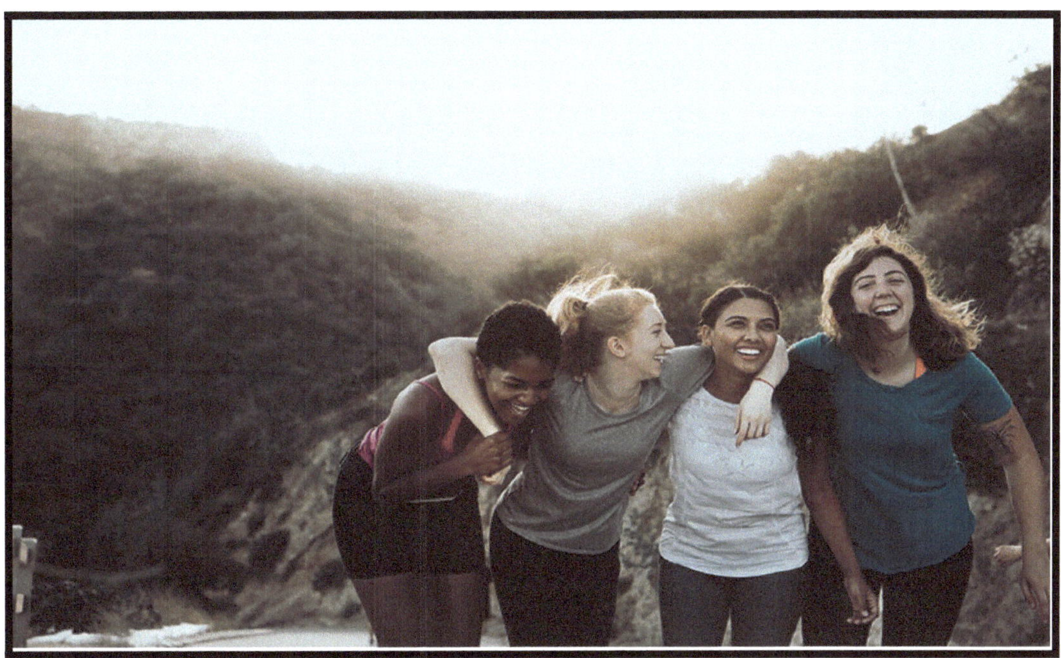

2. Reverse Type 2 Diabetes

This might surprise you, but by being on the ketogenic diet you have the ability to regulate your blood sugar levels. Some people have even been able to reverse their condition completely.

Even if you don't have type 2 diabetes, you can prevent the disease by simply being on the ketogenic diet.

3. Mental Focus

When you are in a state of ketosis, the brain will function on an effective fuel called ketones.

People often experience increased energy when in ketosis which gives you more focus and concentration as the ketones are constantly flowing to the brain throughout the time you are in ketosis.

4. Endurance

When your body uses carbohydrates for energy, this will only last for a couple of hours. *However, your fat stores contain enough energy to last you a few weeks or even months.*

In a state of ketosis, your body will have access to the energy that your fat stores can provide. FINALLY, you're now able to effectively target the stubborn fat that you just couldn't seem to burn off before!

5. Controlling epilepsy

In early 20th century the ketogenic diet was used on children to control epilepsy. It was so successful that adults today are using it to control epilepsy without the use of drugs.

There are many more benefits, but these are a few of the reasons why people want to go on the diet.

Insulin VS Ketosis?

There are many factors that can prevent ketosis, but the most common cause is the presence of insulin.

When you're in the state of ketosis, ketones are used for energy, instead of fat and carbohydrates.

Insulin prevents ketones from being produced and the quickest way to reduce insulin is by watching what you eat.

There are two foods that you should reduce in your diet. They are carbohydrates and protein.

1. Carbohydrates

When you consume carbs, your body will break down the digestible foods into sugar which flows into the blood stream.

Your body then goes into alert mode as it has a high blood sugar level and creates insulin which halts the production of ketones.

Less carbs results in less insulin which translates to more ketones and faster fat loss. It is that simple.

2. Protein

Did you know that excessive protein intake can spike the insulin levels in your body? Not a lot of people are aware of this.

A moderate intake of protein is essential to achieving stable blood sugar levels and providing the body with just enough protein to function optimally.

The keto diet is a fat-based one. The belief is that you need to eat fat to lose fat. When your body is getting copious amounts of fat in its diet, it will be more motivated to shed the fat it's clinging on to.

The body realizes that it has access to ample fuel. So, it doesn't need to store too much for self-preservation.

By cutting down your carb and protein intake, you'll be reducing the amount of insulin in your system greatly. This will help your body set the stage for accelerated weight loss.

The lower the amount of insulin the body produces the better chance that ketones will be created, and you will have no problem getting into ketosis.

Ketosis VS Ketoacidosis

They are two metabolic states the body goes into.

1. Ketosis being the natural way of creating ketones.

2. Ketoacidosis is usually seen in people with type 1 diabetes. It's a state where your body creates ketones at an alarming rate which can turn the blood acidic.

If you can produce insulin, then are you not diabetic and it will be less likely that you will never get into ketoacidosis.

Keto-Adaption

Do you remember the first time you learned how to ride a bike? You kept falling over and over until you mastered the feat of cycling without any problems.

Your body adapts to the keto diet in a similar manner. It has to learn how to create ketones which gives you the fuel you need to carry on with your day to day activities.

This is beginning of what we call keto-adaption.

For someone who is not yet on the keto diet, your body will carry on burning glucose and storing fat. It will take a while for it to adapt and start burning fat instead of glucose for energy.

The entire process can take anywhere from 4 days to a few weeks. How fast your body adapts depends on your current diet.

If you've been on a poor diet that used to be high in sugar, carbs and processed foods, you may experience symptoms such as fatigue and weakness.

These symptoms are normal and as someone who is new to going though keto-adaption, you may have the urge to give up.

Do NOT quit.

To become keto-adapted you need to train your body by consuming less and less foods which are high in sugar and carbohydrates and consume healthy fats such as MCT oil, coconut oil, grass-fed butter and grass-fed meat.

Don't just give up the foods right away. You'll begin to feel ill and weak. This situation is usually referred to as the 'keto flu'.

Your body is cleansing itself. You're probably experiencing sugar cravings or caffeine withdrawal or carb cravings. You're like a drug addict who can't get a fix.

Once you break through these 'addictions' (and that's exactly what they are), your body will feel much better and 'lighter'. Carbohydrates, caffeine and sugar are highly addictive.

You will need some time to get over them.

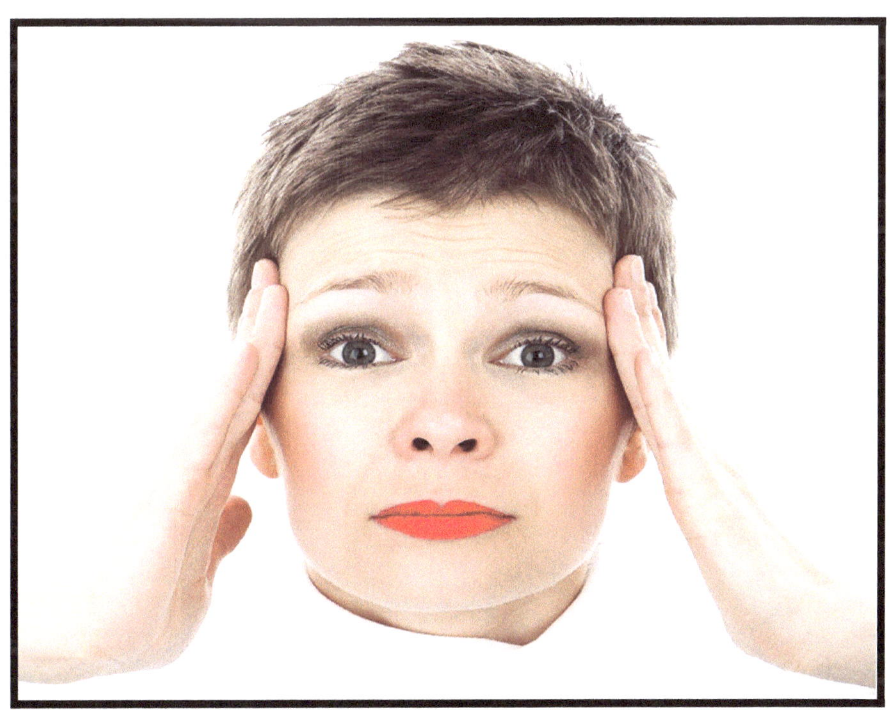

The 'cold turkey' can take a few days or up to a few weeks. So, how can you tell that you're fat adapted.

You need to ask yourself 3 questions:

1. What is the length of time you are going between meals?

If you used to eat every three hours and now you find you can go 6 hours without eating, then you are fat-adapted.

2. Are you feeling motivated and feel full of energy throughout the day?

If you are fat-adapted, then you will have an unlimited supply of energy.

3. Has exercising become easier?

Once you have become adapted to the keto diet, you'll have all the energy you need to keep on exercising.

If you're saying yes to the questions above, then it is highly likely that you are fat-adapted.

Achieving Ketosis

You are ready, primed and about to take the next step into getting into ketosis.

Now, I previously mentioned that you can get into ketosis between a few days to a few weeks, this all depends on you and your body.

How to Quickly Achieve Ketosis?

Here are five steps you can take to speed up the process.

1. Cut carbs slowly.

The recommended amount of carbs to consume while on a keto diet is 30 grams a day. So, try and aim for at least that.

Some may argue that you need to do this gradually to make life easier. But if your goal is to get into ketosis right away then start limiting the carbs you eat today.

2. Increase your fat intake

There are healthy fats and unhealthy fats; you need to consume around 75% of healthy fats as calories.

Foods such as MCT oil or powder, avocado oil, avocados and coconut butter all contribute to healthy fat intake.

3. Intermittent fasting

Fasting is used by a lot of people for a variety of health and religious reasons. It has a range of benefits such as increased energy, low blood sugar levels, faster weight loss and more focus.

If the thought of intermittent fasting scares you, then you may want to try eating around 1200 calories with 80% coming from the fats we talked about above.

4. Exercise

Let's be real here. You need to exercise. Your body requires exercise for it to be healthy and function optimally.

The benefits of regular exercise are so extensive that you just can't be healthy without exercise. Yes, the keto diet WILL help you to lose weight… but weight loss is not the be-all and end-all of good health.

Exercise will strengthen your bones, prevent cardiovascular disease, lower your cholesterol levels, keep you mobile well into your senior years and much more.

Combine your keto diet with regular exercise and not only will you accelerate your weight loss, but you'll be fitter, stronger and have a body that looks fantastic.

5. Make healthy swaps

Starting the keto diet doesn't mean you have to put life on hold, you don't have to stop going out with friends and family.

You can simply make healthy swaps such as:

- No sugar beverages
- Removing dressing from salads
- Having burgers without the bun

These pointers in this chapter will see you into ketosis much faster. It may be hard at first but stick with it and you will start to see and feel the benefits in no time at all.

Foods to Avoid

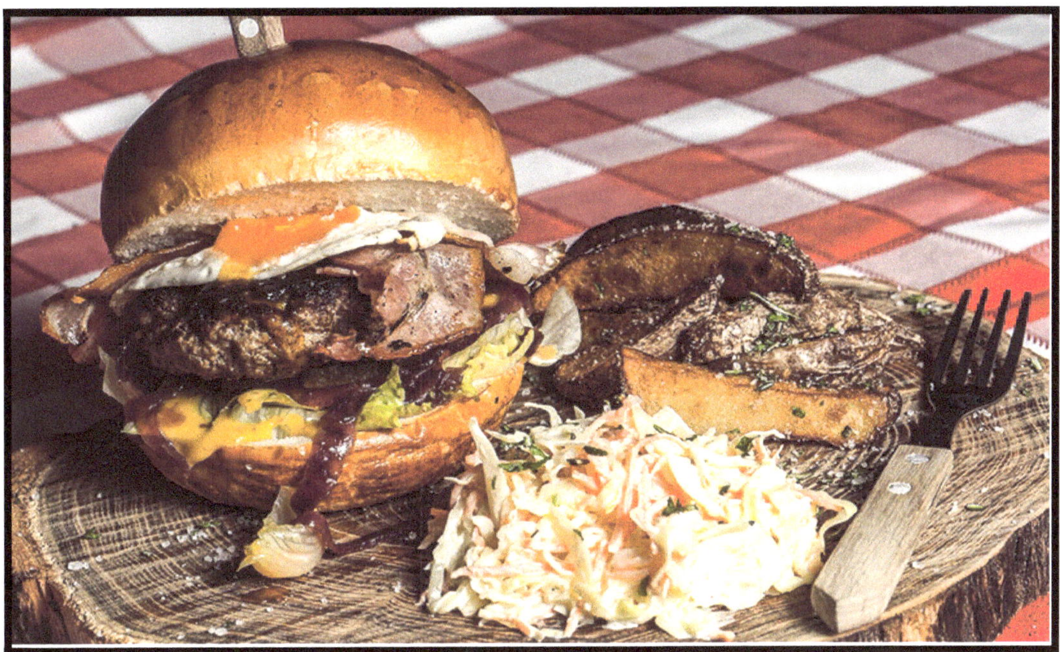

You may think that you know everything there is about what foods you can and cannot eat. However, there are several foods that pass the keto test, but are not quite there yet.

They look good, but in reality, they're not in alignment with the keto diet. Let's look at these 'suspicious' foods and why you should avoid them.

1. **Mayonnaise** – This contains vegetable oil which contains a lot of unhealthy fats.

2. **Chicken** – It just doesn't contain enough fat because it is a lean meat. If you are going to eat chicken, then eat chicken wings as they contain some fat.

3. **Sugar free sweets** – Are they really? When you read the ingredients, you may notice that they may contain maltitol that increases your blood sugar levels. AVOID at all cost!

4. **Salad dressings** – Any dressing that needs contains canola oil, soybean oil, or sunflower oil needs to be avoided.

5. **Vegetables** – For years everyone from your parents to the media have been preaching that veggies are important. That is true, but not all vegetables are suited for the keto diet.

   Avoid root grown vegetables, white potatoes, etc. that contain starch. These will just make you feel bloated.

6. **Nuts** – Nuts are high in omega-6 which is what we don't want in our diet so try and stick to macadamia and pecan nuts.

Exercising While on the Keto Diet

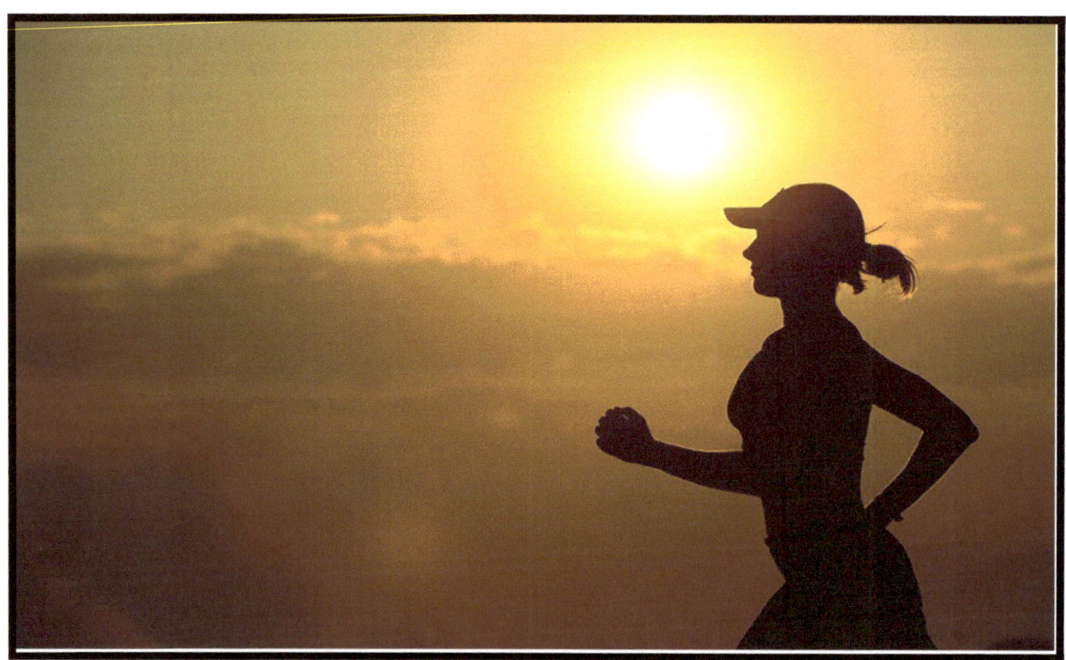

When you are in ketosis, you'll be restricting your carb intake. This will stop your muscles from accessing sugar which your body heavily relies on.

When your muscles don't have enough fuel (glucose in this case) the ability for them to handle high intensity exercise is limited.

Any high intensity exercise over 10 seconds should be avoided. You do not need hard exercise to lose weight. The keto diet is so powerful that the fat will still melt off.

You may engage in activities such as walking, swimming, cycling, etc. As long as you maintain a moderate pace, you'll not be taxing your body. Weight training is great too. Just don't overdo it.

Low intensity aerobic exercises are great. So are yoga and Pilates sessions. Stability exercises are good too.

Once you're fully keto-adapted, you can progress on to higher-intensity training. It's always during the initial stages when you have to be most careful

As mentioned earlier, Tyson Fury who was prepping for his fight in December 2018 was consuming 5500 calories a day but exercising non-stop. He still lost 140 pounds and became fighting fit.

The keto diet and exercising can really drop the weight off. If you feel dizzy or something is not right, stop and assess your situation. If needed, seek professional medical advice.

What to Expect When Going into Ketosis?

The ketogenic diet is without a doubt the most popular way to lose weight and when followed correctly, your ketone levels will rise, and your insulin levels will drop.

However, it is still hard to tell when you are in ketosis.

Here are common positive and negative signs that can help you identify if you are in ketosis.

1. Weight loss

You will almost immediately drop a lot of weight due to water being flushed out your system and then gradually your weight will decrease.

2. Bad breath

This is a good sign as once you have bad breath you would have nearly reached full ketosis.

If this is affecting your social life, then you may want to chew on some sugar free gum – just be sure to check the labels for carbohydrates as they do digest into sugar.

3. Increased ketone levels

As you continue the keto diet, you'll have an increase in ketone levels and the best way to measure this is via a test kit. You want to be in a range of 0.5–3.0 mmol/L.

4. Low Appetite

Not feeling as hungry and sometimes skipping meals is a good sign as ketones are sending signals to your brain to reduce your appetite.

5. Focus and Energy

When you start the keto diet, you will feel weak but as you start to get more energy and focus, you know you are on the right track.

6. Digestive issues

For the first few days at the start of your diet you may experience constipation and diarrhea. Eating low carb vegetables that are high in fiber will help ease your stomach.

7. Insomnia

When you change your diet, you may find it difficult to sleep as your body is adapting to the changes and craving for carbohydrates or it is hungry. This problem will gradually disappear in a week or two.

These are signs and symptoms you can keep an eye on but if you are losing weight gradually then there is no need to monitor your ketone levels every single day.

Dealing with Keto Flu

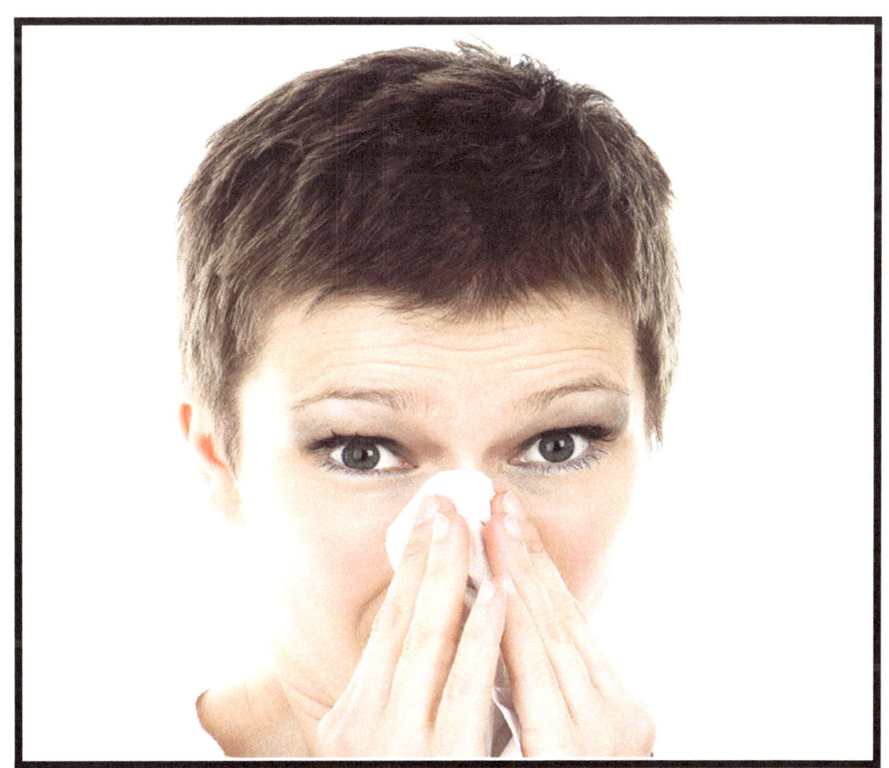

You may have experienced the flu at some time in your life and the keto flu is no different. These similar symptoms are caused by reducing the intake of carbohydrates.

By reducing the amount of carbohydrates your body will start to burn ketones for energy.

This quick change in your body will come a shock to the system and cause withdrawal symptoms.

Switching to the keto diet is a big change and your body will need time to adapt to this way of eating.

Symptoms will be different from person to person and some may not experience anything at all, but here are some common issues you may face:

- Nausea and Vomiting
- Constipation and Diarrhea
- Poor concentration
- Stomach pain
- Muscle soreness
- Insomnia
- Cravings
- Headaches

Keto-flu is temporary, however there are a few things you can do to limit or even completely get rid of symptoms.

1. Drink plenty of water

When you begin your diet, you'll lose a lot of water so drinking plenty of water will keep you hydrated. Drink often and drink throughout the day.

2. Replenish electrolytes

Your electrolytes will be out of balance and you can restore balance by increasing your salt intake and eating foods high in potassium such as salmon, avocados and nuts. Some people have a tin of sardines as it is high in calcium.

3. Exercise

In the beginning stages of keto flu, you may not feel like doing the exercise you were used to doing. So, keep it low-key for the first few weeks with light exercise twice a week.

4. Increase fats

Your body is now on a very low-carb diet. So, increasing the good fats as a fuel source is must. Add a little MCT oil in your coffee which will bump up the amount of fat you are allowed.

5. Take exogenous ketones

Adding more ketones to your body will help you overcome ketosis more quickly. Exogenous ketones come in the form of supplements.

By using the tips above, you'll be available to avoid most of these symptoms all together.

Measuring Ketosis

Now we get to the fun part…

We are going to cover how ketones are measured and different ways on how to measure them.

Is the very first chapter we spoke about the three types of ketones that your body will produce which are Acetone, Acetoacetate and Beta-Hydroxybutyrate (BHB for short). Each of these ketones are tested in their own way.

- Acetone ketone is tested via breath
- BHB is tested via the blood stream
- Acetoacetate is tested via urine

Why Measuring Ketosis Can Help?

Anyone can measure their weight to see if their diet is working, but measuring ketosis is a much better alternative.

Monitoring your keto levels is vital to staying on track on your keto diet. By knowing exactly what your levels are, you'll be able to adjust your diet and routine accordingly.

Your weight can increase or decrease throughout the day but by knowing the level of ketones you have in your body, you'll be able to find out if you are burning fat.

Some people may be building muscle by reducing fat. Since the scales can only show weight gain or weight loss using numbers that can be misleading as you don't know what the numbers represent. Because muscle weighs more than fat, the increase in numbers on the scale could be from muscle and not fat.

By measuring ketosis, you can see if you're actually getting rid of body fat.

To be in a fat-burning state, you need to aim for levels of between 1.5 to 3.0 mmol/l and there are three ways you can measure this.

1. Keto Strips/Sticks

Most people on the ketogenic diet will prefer to use keto strips which are measured using urine (acetoacetate).

The reason being is they are cheap, and you can pick them up from Amazon for around $8 for 100 strips. The downside to the cheaper option is that it can be inaccurate.

They are inaccurate due to the fact that before going on the keto diet or just as you're starting the diet the body, it with naturally pass more ketones.

Once you have adapted to ketosis and got past the keto-flu stage then it will be an ideal time to use keto strips.

Once opened keto sticks/strips usually last three months and as there are 100 strips depending on which pack you buy, you can test twice a day - once in the morning and once in the evening a few hours after a meal.

2. Keto Breathalyzer

A keto breathalyzer also called a ketonix is a handheld device that measures acetone ketones in your breath and the results are in real time.

It works like an alcohol breathalyzer. You blow into in the ketonix and it will give you a reading, which you match against its unique chart to see how far into ketosis are.

You can test yourself using a ketonix at any time and one of the advantages is that you can use it anywhere.

The costs for one can start at $20 and can go all the way up to $250. It all depends on quality.

Go with one that suits your budget and know that you usually get what you pay for. So, it's better to get the slightly more expensive ones that are more accurate and with more features.

3. Blood Ketometer

This ketometer measures Beta-hydroxybutyrate (BHB) and has proven to be the most accurate method of checking your ketone levels. By using a little drop of your blood, you'll have a precise reading in a matter of seconds.

Some meters do come with a lancet pen and a supply of strips included, but if they don't then you can get them at a very low cost.

Prick your finger with the pen, drop a little blood on the strip and let it absorb well. The meter will then give you a reading.

The four sets of universal readings you need to work from are:

1. Less than 1.0 mmol/L – Not in ketosis
2. Between 1.0 and 1.5 mmol/L – In ketosis but not on the keto diet
3. 1.5 and 3.0 mmol/L – Optimal ketosis
4. 3.0 mmol/L and above – Unhealthy levels of ketones

Blood ketone meters are more accurate than the other keto strips and breathalyzer as you are testing the source and not just a by-product like acetones.

If you're taking supplements, the results will not be affected in the readings either.

The only disadvantage is that blood meters are expensive and the strips need to be replaced.

If you are losing weight via the keto diet, then a blood ketometer is probably not required. However, if you're competing in a sport or have clients that are, then it would be a good investment.

Measuring your ketone levels is important if you want to lose weight quickly and effectively. If you're looking to only lose a few pounds, then there's no need to invest in expensive tests.

Intermittent Fasting

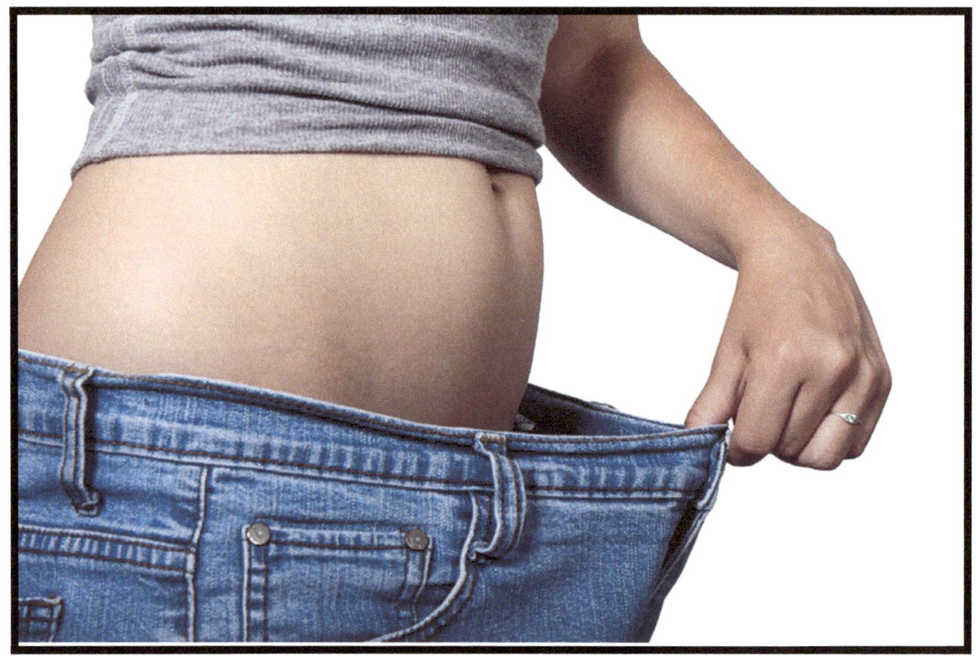

Intermittent fasting is a great way to slim down, become more focused and stay fit without changing the way you've been eating or even changing the diet you are currently on.

When you're intermittent fasting, you will eat much less because your appetite will decrease over time. It is great option for those that want to reduce the number of calories you consume.

You fast by only eating during a specified duration (eating window) which can last anywhere from 5 to 8 hours. Any other time outside this window will mean that you're fasting and can't eat anything.

There are two basic protocols that people work from - the 16/8 protocol, where you fast for 16 hours and eat during an 8-hour window... or the 24-hour protocol where you don't eat for 24 hours.

There are people who have lost up to 12 pounds just by fasting. While a lot of it will be water weight, you would have lost quite a bit of fat too.

For the remainder of this chapter we will refer to intermittent fasting as IF.

Benefits of Intermittent Fasting

Besides losing weight, IF does come with the following benefits.

- *Insulin levels drop* – During ketosis there is a low level of insulin in your blood. This results in fat burning. Couple this with IF and you are a walking, talking fat-burning machine.

- *Weight loss* – When you're in a fasted state, you'll notice that your stomach "shrinks", which results in you eating less and losing more fat.

- *Lower risk of Type 2 Diabetes* – As your insulin decreases due to IF, it will also lower your blood sugar levels. IF has been used in clinical studies which have proven this to be true.

- *Reduce Stress* – Not just any stress but oxidative stress which causes aging. People who fast intermittently look younger.

- *Healthy Heart* – IF can reduce risks for heart disease such as cholesterol and blood pressure.

- *Activate cellular repair* – Your body begins to dump a lot of waste including water and starts to repair itself.

- *Fights cancer* – Fasting can slow down the growth of cancer cells and even stop cancer from taking root in your body.

These benefits are only scratching the surface as to what can be achieved with intermittent fasting.

Combining Intermittent Fasting with Keto

You have begun your keto diet.

You are starting to lose a little weight, but it's not fast enough.

What can you do to improve it?

Intermittent fasting and KETO. That's what.

Intermittent fasting and keto are two separate strategies to lose weight. Both methods produce enough ketones to burn body fat.

Intermittent fasting and keto work towards the same goal which is achieving ketosis. So, the question many people ask is, "Why not stick to just one?"

The answer is quite simple.

The keto diet receives a long-term boost when combined with intermittent fasting. IF becomes a lot more effective when used in conjunction with the keto diet.

It's a win-win situation.

You won't feel as hungry when combining the two, and since you're fasting there will be no crashes due to the lack of sugar.

Intermittent fasting while on the keto diet works!

How to Start Intermittent Fasting?

Embarking on the keto diet can be intimidating. There are cases where people are afraid to get started due to fear and mindset issues.

Before you start, you need to have clear and concise goals for yourself. Do you want to:

1. Lose weight?
2. Prevent diseases?

3. Live longer?

You need to set aside worries and common misconceptions such as eating fatty foods will make you fat, or that breakfast is the most important meal of the day.

These outdated beliefs are halting your weight loss progress. Give yourself a chance to try something new and amazing. You'll never look back.

Here's a quick challenge that you can try.

> **Day 1:** Make you last dinner around 7pm and then drink water till you go to bed.
>
> **Day 2:** You are awake at 7pm, delay that breakfast till at least 10am then carry about your day.
>
> **Day 3:** Same again don't eat until 10am, eat lunch and don't eat anything until dinner at around 7pm.
>
> **Day 4:** Skip breakfast but have lunch at 11am so you will be going 16hrs without food. Don't have any snacks and eat dinner at 7pm.
>
> **Day 5:** Repeat day 4 again. Congratulations you have gone through a quick 5 day fast.

Use this 5-day challenge to get a feel for intermittent fasting. You may even see results in this short time.

However, with intermittent fasting will come the downsides such as fatigue and brain fog which are similar to that of keto flu. Therefore, before you begin make sure:

1. You seek medical advice before you start.
2. Keep it simple and easy.
3. Follow a schedule that suits you. You don't have to have a last meal at 7pm.

Overall intermittent fasting will allow you to lose weight and improve your health over the long run.

What is Allowed During Fasting?

Common sense says that you should not eat at all during your fasting window. While you are fasting…do not consume any calories. It's as simple as that.

You are allowed something to drink as you need to stay hydrated throughout your fasting. However, your drinks should contain no calories.

Here are few options:

1. **Water** – You can drink water all day long, but avoid adding any cordial to it. You can add a squeeze of lime to give it a bit of taste to make things a little different.

2. **Coffee** – Black coffee is all you can drink. Adding a little cream or milk is a big no. Remember to drink it slowly as you may upset your stomach.

3. **Broths** – Don't buy any broths from your local market. Instead, make one at home. Nothing is better than homemade and stick to vegetable broths.

4. **Tea** – Any tea is fine but green tea is the best as it helps suppress your appetite.

5. **Apple Cider Vinegar** – It helps regulate your blood sugar levels and makes intermittent fasting work a lot better.

Again, just keep it stupidly simple. Don't drink or eat anything with calories while you are in your fasting window and you are golden.

Getting Maximum Benefits

There are several ways you can get started with intermittent fasting, and we suggest that you get started with a fast that is easy for you.

Here are a few options to choose from:

1. **12 hours fast** – You need to decide when you want to start. The most popular is to fast between 7pm till 7am the next morning.

2. **16 hours fast** - Same as the 12 hours fast, but you may be skipping breakfast or lunch.

3. **2 day fast** - Eat for 5 days and reduce your calorie intake for 2 days. Don't stop eating for 2 days. Simply consume less calories. Around 500 calories is safe.

4. **Alternate fasting** – For a quick loss in weight, try alternate fasting and only consume around 500 calories during your fasting days. Don't try alternative fasting if you are beginner.

5. **24 fast once a week** – You don't consume anything during this fast for around 1 to 2 days. Be careful on this fast as it can cause you headaches.

Your experience and requirements are different from everyone else. Decide for yourself which is the best fast for you.

Make sure you stay hydrated throughout your fast by drinking plenty of water throughout the day and you can have the occasional green tea.

Relax as much as you can while enjoying light exercise or a gentle walk, just don't become a coach potato.

Count your calories and don't go over the recommended allowance during fasting days where you are consuming around 500 per day. This is based on your activity levels.

For the absolute best results on non-fasting days, eat a healthy meal.

Quickest Way to Achieve Ketosis

Ketosis is a natural way of your body producing more ketones to burn off fat and allows you to stay fit and healthy.

A lot of people are turning to the keto diet as a way to lose weight but the weight loss only starts when you are in ketosis.

The main question people have is *"What is the quickest way I can get into ketosis?"*

We are going to give you a few tips as well as little more information about protein, exogenous ketones, bullet proof coffee and much more.

To help you get into ketosis a lot quicker, we have compiled a list to assist you:

1. Eat more healthy fat by eating foods that contain coconut oil, avocado oil and butter.

2. Supplements can help you get into ketosis in as quick as 24hrs which will touch on in the next chapter.

3. Eat fewer carbohydrates as your body will begin to turn to burning fat as an energy source opposed to glucose.

4. Consume more MCT – A lot of people on the keto diet, include this in their morning coffee know as bullet proof coffee.

5. Exercise more but keep it light.

6. Eat a balanced amount of protein.

7. Try fasting to speed up the process.

There are many more tips, but these are the main ones to get you into ketosis quickly.

Let's look at a few more points.

What You Need to Know About Protein?

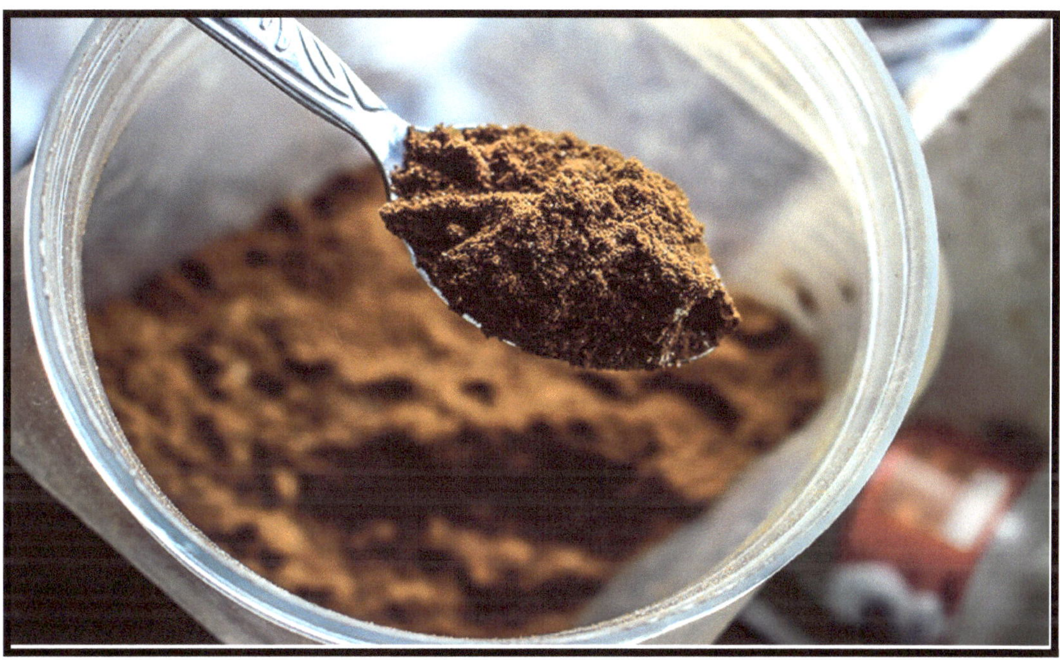

Protein is one nutrient that many people take for granted while on the keto diet. Protein is crucial in any diet as it will have an effect on:

1. **The functionality of the brain**
2. **Health of bones of skin**
3. **Muscle growth**
4. **Recovery after workouts**
5. **Reducing body fat**

The above allows you to live a longer life and boosts your metabolism, but some people worry that too much protein will push you back out of ketosis.

The truth is that protein is crucial to the keto diet, and you should eat enough of it to lose weight as it will replace any new fat coming in to the body.

Remember you want the already stored fat in your body to burn first.

Protein contains fewer calories than fat. If you do not consume protein as part of your diet you can suffer from weak muscles, sluggish brain activity, a compromised immune system and your risk of disease will increase.

You're probably asking yourself right now – *"How much protein do I need?"*

The amount required may vary from person to person, but if you are not as active as you were in your teens it is recommended to consume around 0.8 grams of protein per pound of body mass.

If you are very active or training for a sporting event then consume 1-1.2 grams of protein per pound of bodyweight.

Don't be afraid of adding protein to your diet. Just don't add too much of it. Testing yourself to see if you're in ketosis will help keep you on track.

Exogenous Ketones

Not everyone will burn the same amount of fat even if they're on the exact same diet and training regimen. There are many factors in play and people are different.

Ultimately, achieving your best with the keto diet will boil down to how much ketones your body is producing. If your body's production of ketones is low, consuming exogenous ketones will be perfect to give you the boost you need.

Exogenous ketones are a supplement which is directly sent to the cells for energy whereas the body would burn fats, transport nutrients to the liver and turn them into ketones.

Exogenous ketones are like an instant hit. They can be found in a variety of products such as salts, oils and raw ketone esters and can be used:

1. **To burn fat** – Using exogenous ketones will tell your body to start using ketones for energy which will then result in fat being burned.

2. **Get into ketosis sooner** – Once you're in ketosis it is very easy to fall out of it and very hard to get back into it. ½ scoop of exogenous ketones will get you back into ketosis within 24hrs.

3. **Assist you with keto-flu** – Your body will go into a state of shock when you transition into ketosis. Less than half a scoop will ease that transition period.

4. **Increase in endurance** – If you need energy right away, rather than burning fat, exogenous ketones will provide that instant energy for you. It is commonly used by athletes.

If you are struggling to get into ketosis then I would recommend exogenous ketones.

Bullet Proof Coffee

If you are like one of those high impact, high performing people that need their bit off coffee every morning or if you simply need that extra amount of good fat – bullet proof coffee is your answer.

It literally stops you from craving food and is completely replaced as a meal and doesn't give you the negative effects that caffeine does.

It will also help you increase focus and performance and it contains MCT oil which is crucial as it contains good fats which helps with weight loss.

Ingredients needed for bullet proof coffee.

- 1 cup of hot coffee

- 1tbsp of grass fed/unsalted butter
- 1tbsp of MCT oil

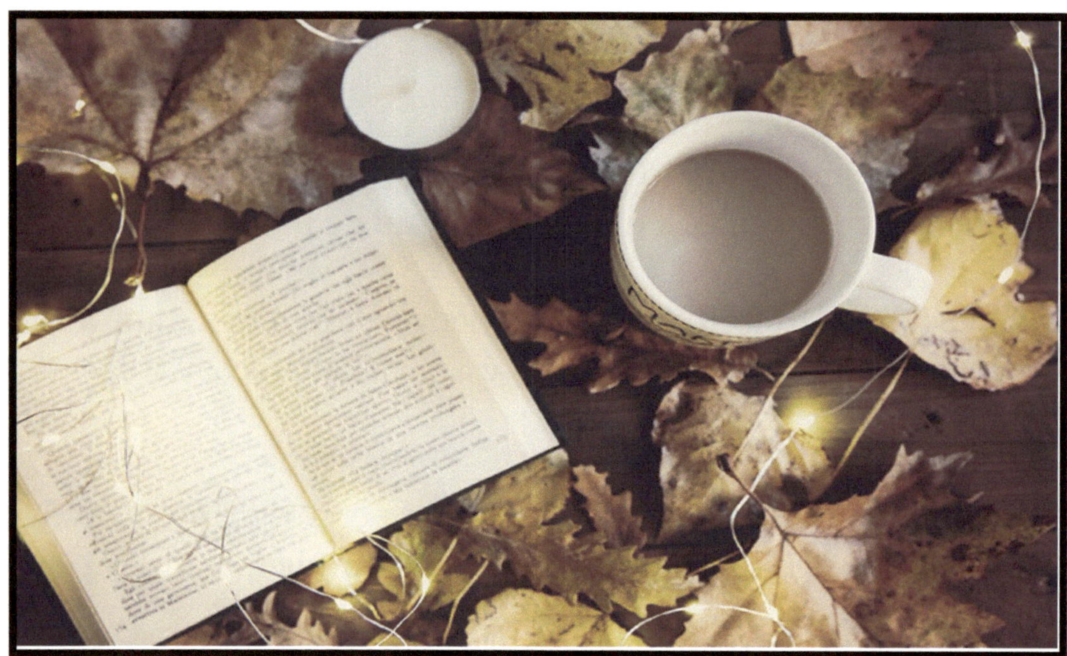

Put all the ingredients in a blender and enjoy your new morning ritual as it comes with positive health benefits unlike the usual latte.

Hidden Sugars

So, you can read the labels and point out carbs in every type of food but something that you often scan past is hidden sugar.

If you are not careful with what you eat, then you may be taking on more sugar than you should.

When a label says no sugar, you need to take extra care as to what is actually in it. If any label says no sugar or no refined sugar, then there will be alternatives used in the production of that food.

There aren't just a few sugar alternatives out there; there are in fact hundreds such as:

- Invert sugar
- Brown sugar
- Honey
- Malt syrup
- Maple syrup
- Raw sugar

The bolder the statement of no sugar is on the ingredients label, the more careful you need to be.

Ingredients such as Mannitol, Maltitol, Sorbitol, Splenda, Isomalt and lactitol contain sugar or cause insulin spikes and need to be avoided at all cost.

You can find these types of sugars in sugar free drinks, protein bars, store bought green smoothies, non-dairy milks and salad dressing.

Keep an eye on the labels, keep your carbs to the minimum and you'll be hitting ketosis quite quickly.

Fats You Need to Avoid

There are good fats and bad fats. Bad fats are trans-fats or some other fat that's detrimental to your body. The hydrogenated vegetable oils sold in supermarkets are NOT good for your health.

When you go grocery shopping, make sure you avoid:

- Vegetable oils such as corn, vegetable, safflower and canola.
- Margarine and Vegetable shortening

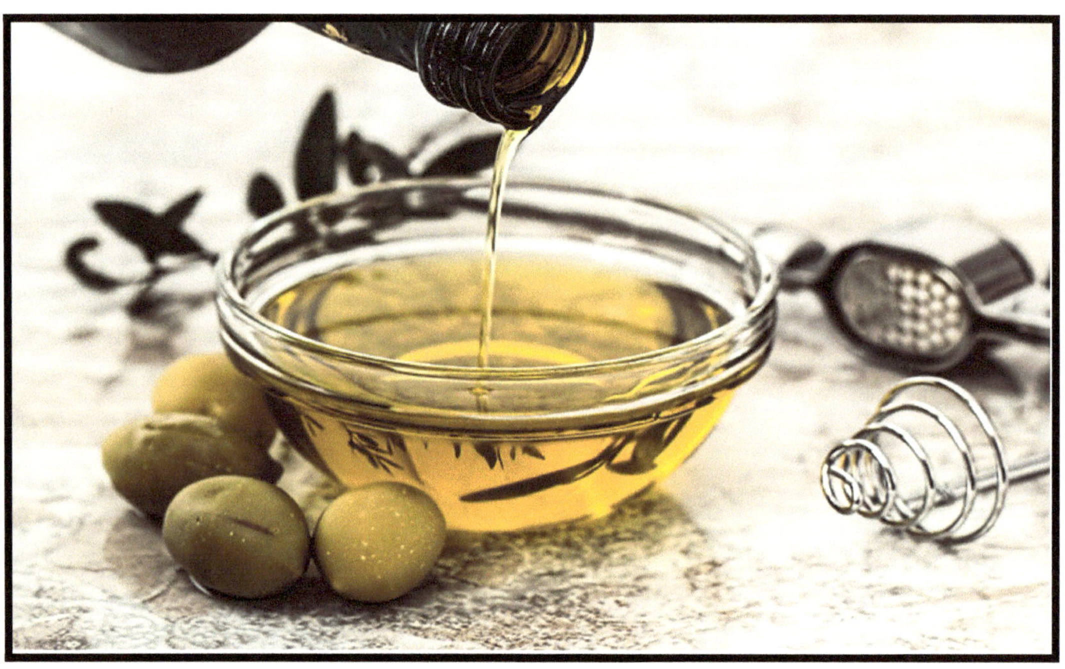

Avoiding Alcohol

You don't have to avoid alcohol all the time. Just make sure it's not a daily habit.

When you drink alcohol, you'll begin to feel hungry and this can cause you to eat junk food which will kick you out of ketosis quite quickly. Not only that, lager contains a huge number of calories so stay clear.

Alcohol is toxic to your body and your body reacts in such a way that it stops burning your fat and turns its attention to getting rid of alcohol.

If you are on a keto diet and have a party night with beer and wine, be ready to suffer in the morning. You will get drunk a lot faster as well suffer the worst hangover.

If you are new to the keto diet, the best advice is to avoid alcohol altogether especially if you are looking to lose weight.

Supplements

Using supplements while on the ketogenic diet can make your progression from start to ketosis a breeze as well as provide you the nutrients you're missing from traditional foods.

For the ketogenic diet to work, you need to understand supplements. Your body is going through a change where it breaks down carbs in glucose to burning fat from your fat stores.

Supplements also help you overcome:

1. Keto-flu

The transition can be hard and keto-flu is common for people who don't use vitamins or minerals. As your body burns the remainder of glucose in your body, water is lost and with-it important electrolytes.

2. Nutritional gaps

You are restricted to certain foods when on the keto diet such as fruit and vegetables that contain starch. Supplements such as greens tablets will give you the nutrients you need, as your body gets used to only eating red meat and eggs.

3. Health goals

Have you set yourself certain health goals while on the keto diet? Supplements can help. If you want more weight loss, take a spoonful of MCT oil.

Understanding what each supplement can do for you will help you achieve your goals.

The Best Supplements

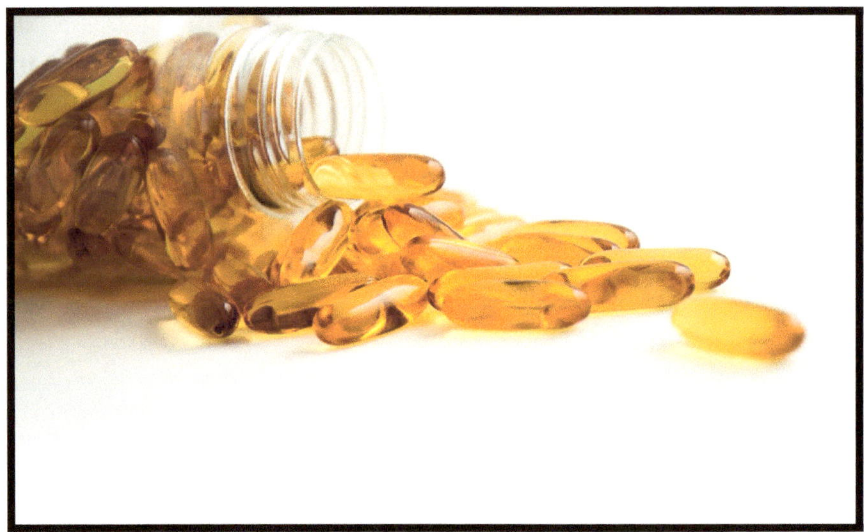

Not all supplements are made equal. There are some which are perfect for keto and some which you need avoid.

1. Vitamin D

When you are in ketosis and lack vitamin D you can suffer weakness, muscle breakdown, weak bone density.

If you live a sunny place, then exposure to sun will give you all the vitamin D you need. The safer option would be to eat fatty fish or 400 IU tablets per day.

2. MCT oil

It is a type of fat that can give the body energy almost immediately. It creates ketones quickly and puts you in ketosis very quickly.

It helps by keeping you in the metabolic state of burning fat without you worrying if you are going to fall out of ketosis.

You can find MCT oil in butter, yogurt, cheese, coconut oil but the majority of people use MCT oil and have it with their coffee as we mentioned in earlier chapters.

3. Electrolytes

The important ones such as sodium, magnesium, calcium and potassium. Now you are going to get all these from the keto diet but just not enough.

Sodium you get from Himalayan salt, bone broth and red meat. Be careful with how much you do take. ¾ of a teaspoon is safe enough.

Magnesium can be found in spinach, avocado and mackerel. You can also buy magnesium tablets from your local store and around 400mg per day is adequate.

Potassium helps break down carbs and build proteins. It can be found in avocados, salmon, and mushrooms.

Calcium makes sure your bones stay strong and reduces blood clotting. Calcium can be found in dairy products such as milk but that is something we want to avoid on the keto diet. You can purchase calcium tablets and the recommendation is around 1000mg per day.

4. Omega-3 Fatty Acids (fish oil supplements)

This supplement is extremely powerful and should be used by everyone even if they're not on a keto diet. Our diets these days are out of whack with too much omega-6 fatty acids being consumed and not enough omega-3s.

As a result, inflammation arises and many diseases start to creep in. Omega-3 fish oils help to lower your risk of heart disease and it is a fatty acid which is perfect for the keto diet. It can be found in salmon, sardines and anchovies.

5. Digestive Enzymes

These are useful for helping you transition into the keto diet and it prevents nausea and diarrhea.

Exogenous ketones

As previously mentioned, you can use these to get you into ketosis quickly and supply you with a quick boost of energy.

6. Greens powder

This supplement provides a means for you to get your daily intake of vegetables. They contain extract from plants like spirulina, chlorella, kale and broccoli.

The ketogenic diet can provide everything you absolutely need to fill in your nutritional voids. However, we are human and can't stay on track all time.

The supplements above will help you stay in ketosis without sacrificing the nutrients your body needs.

Conclusion

You've made it this far and are ready to start on the keto diet.

Initially, it will be tough to adapt to and you'll have to endure the keto flu for the first few days. Don't lose hope. If you stick with it, the symptoms will pass.

Here are a few tips that will help you on your way if you get stuck.

Pick a day and start your keto diet by limiting the amount of carbs you consume so that glucose levels drop greatly, and your body starts to burn fat for energy.

As soon as you can, head to your local health store and grab some MCT oil, use the recipe for bullet proof coffee and have that first thing in the morning to give you more focus to stay on track on your diet.

Get rid of any remaining glucose in your body by exercising a little. A brisk 15-minute walk is all you need to jump start your body to producing ketones.

The keto diet is all about good fats. We covered a whole lot about good fats and the best one. Get your fridge stocked today.

Combine intermittent fasting as soon as you can for quick results. The first week you have experienced a huge loss in weight due to water drop.

Start with a simple fast of only eating between 10am and 7pm. Drink green tea in between.

Consume protein is small amounts only. Don't starve yourself of every nutrient. Re-visit the supplements chapter for quick recap.

Buy keto strips from Amazon or your local health store and test yourself and test yourself each day to see where you are and adjust where needed.

What to Do If You Cannot Fast Intermittently?

You and your friends started intermittent fasting together. However, only friends are seeing the benefits and have lost 10lbs.

You on the other hand haven't seen any progress, and it could be down to one or more reasons.

1. **Starting right away** – Jumping into intermittent fasting is just the same as jumping into a pit of fire. You are clearly going to fail. If you're eating every couple of hours it will be harder to start eating every 6 hours. Start with a 12 hour fast two weeks into keto and you will be fine.

2. **Not planning correctly** – Your window and fasting times are different from everyone else. If you work nights and don't eat from 7pm till 7am, you will burn out. Instead fast when you get home till you go back to work the next day.

3. **Eat during your window** – If you are not eating what you are supposed to eat during you window, you may put on more weight instead. Your window is your window so eat when you are hungry.

4. **Look out for what you eat** – Your window is your window but keep an eye on what you eat. Fasting doesn't mean you need to take a trip down McDonalds, instead look at what foods you are allowed to eat as part of your keto diet.

5. **Dehydration** – Intermittent fasting is about not consuming calories during your fasting window. This doesn't mean you should stop drinking water. Make sure you keep yourself hydrated with enough water.

You will at times feel the hunger creeping in. Acknowledge it and occupy yourself with something else to do besides eating.

After a while, the hunger will pass. Usually, people get hungry around the times that they're used to eating. Once you've passed that time, the hunger will dissipate and only return later.

It always comes in waves. So, just aim to get over the wave… and you'll make it through a few more hours until the next wave. With time, your appetite will decrease, and you'll not have to deal with hunger pangs anymore.

Take the time to build up your fasting windows, let your body get used to it and you will thrive.

Using Keto for Weight Loss

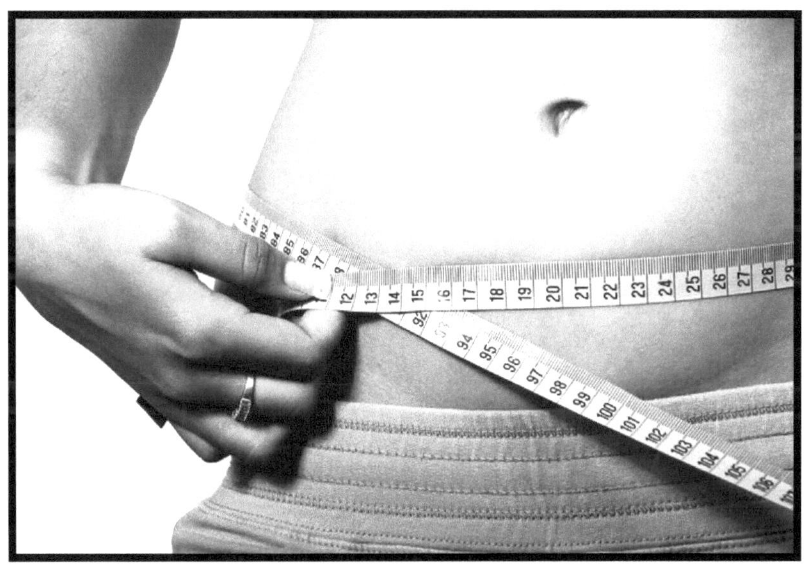

The keto diet is mostly used for weight loss and it will take some longer than others to see the benefits.

There are four factors that determines how much you will lose and in what space of time.

1. **Your current health state** – If you are overweight, resistant to insulin or simply cannot burn fat as fast as the majority of people then you will lose weight a lot slower.

2. **Your body** – What is your BMI? Do you need to burn a lot of fat? In the beginning, if you have a lot of fat to burn you will see some weight loss very quickly, whereas a leaner person make take longer. Over time, the results will taper off.

3. **Current habits** – What is your current diet like? Are you eating keto only foods and reading the labels to make sure you are not taking on hidden sugar? Are you exercising? Changing your habits to positive ones will set you up for success.

4. **Transition into ketosis** – If this is the first time you are on a keto diet, then becoming fat-adapted will take a little longer. Your body needs to learn to product ketones and then use fat as an energy source.

Stay on track by eating the correct amounts of keto food, remember that the keto diet is not just about going on a diet; it is a way of life. So, treat it as your new lifestyle.

During your first week on the keto diet you can expect to lose up to 10 pounds as you are losing water. Just remember to keep drinking more water than usual to avoid become dehydrated.

After two weeks, your body is getting used to creating ketones and the cycle of burning fat starts. It will be steady and consistent. Expect to lose up to 2 pounds per week.

As you progress further into your diet, you will start to see the fat come off and the weight loss slowing down as the calories you are eating is sustaining your current physical needs.

Sit back and re-evaluate what you need to do next to increase the weight loss further.

21-Day Challenge

If you are still unsure of where or how to start, consider signing up for our **21-Day Challenge** at: https://forms.aweber.com/form/88/537832688.htm. Each day of the challenge you will get an email with a task to do for that day and the action steps required to complete it. Here is a sample of Day 1:

==

Day 1 – Goal Setting

To get the result you have always wanted to set clear concise goals of what you want to achieve on your keto diet.

Setting a determined weight loss goal is going to be more difficult that you think as you will need to work it out and it could be more a number of reasons.

This can be anything from losing a few pounds to maybe over 20 lbs., you may want to reverse type 2 diabetes or even lower your cholesterol.

There is no point in taking the wrong steps to reach your desired goal as you will never get there.

Back on to goals, if you goal is weight loss then you need to keep the amount low to begin with something along the lines of 10% loss of your current weight. So, if you are 200 lbs., you want to aim for 20lbs loss which will give you a finish weight of 180lbs.

This is much more achievable than to say you want to lose 64lbs upfront which is ridiculous.

For your first day, don't worry about what you are going to eat or what exercise you will complete that day rather have a look at what is in your cupboards.

Getting rid of all junk food is paramount to seeing results. Look, I have been there myself. You may be able to resist for quite some time, but the hunger does take over.

Action Steps:

Write down what you want to achieve from keto and put it somewhere safe.

Go into your kitchen with an empty box and go through each cupboard and empty of the contents into the box of all non-keto food like chips, chocolates and vegetables.

Look everywhere – inside bigger containers and pots, there is always something lurking around that will take you out of ketosis.

Congratulations you made it through the first day, now dust off those old trainers and go for a 15-minute walk.

==

The keto diet will have different effects on the body for everybody. Listen to your body and make changes as and when you need to.

There are many Facebook groups you can join for tips and peer support. Share your love for the diet, share recipes, learn and ask questions.

You've got this!

About the Author

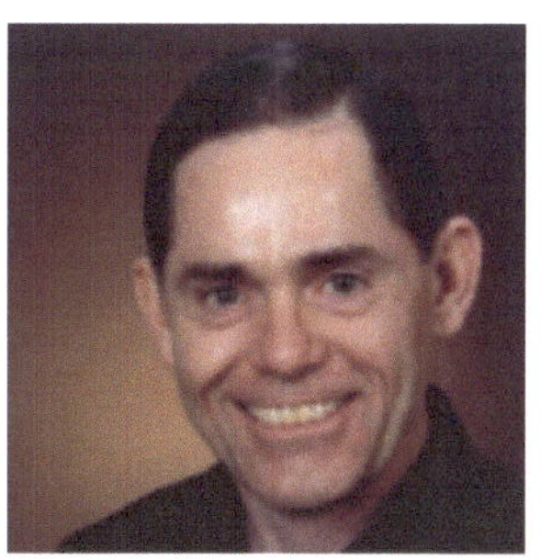

I grew up in Central Minnesota, where my parents owned and operated a fishing resort. Once out of high school I tried a couple of semesters of college, only to quit halfway through the Spring term; I decided at that time that college wasn't for me.

Then I decided to follow my father's previous occupation as an auto mechanic. I graduated from a two-year of vocational training course and worked as a mechanic for five years. While in vocational training, I decided to join the National Guard where I eventually ended up working full-time for 32 years.

So how does all of this relate to writing? In one of my leadership schools, the instructor, who was an English teacher at a juvenile detention center, presented writing to me in a whole new way - a way that started to develop my interest in working with words.

I eventually went back to college on the GI Bill while I was working and earned my Bachelor's degree in Business Administration. Taking a class or two per semester at night and on weekends took me seven years to complete my degree.

Fast forward about 40 years and I now have published over 100 books on Amazon for Kindle, CreateSpace and other publishing platforms.

Besides my own writing, I also ghostwrite ebooks, books, reports, articles, blogs and do Kindle conversions for clients on a variety of topics.

Today my wife and I are retired from our careers and live in Gold Canyon, AZ. I now write as a retirement business where you'll find me happily sitting in my office typing away on my laptop as I work on my next book or ghostwriting project . . . that is if we are not traveling on a cruise ship - our new-found mode of travel.

Thank-you for purchasing this book. If you are interested in purchasing and reading more of my published books, you can go to: https://www.amazon.com/Ron-Kness/e/B0072M6PYO.